STEPS TO RECOVERY:

THRIVING AFTER JOINT REPLACEMENT SURGERY

COPYRIGHT

CONTENTS

INTRODUCTION

Understanding Joint Replacement Surgery:

Joint replacement surgery, whether for the knee, hip, or shoulder, represents a significant medical advancement that has dramatically improved the quality of life for millions of people worldwide. The procedure involves removing the damaged or diseased parts of the joint and replacing them with artificial components, which are designed to mimic the natural function of the joint. The most common reasons for joint replacement are osteoarthritis, rheumatoid arthritis, and traumatic injury, all of which can lead to pain, stiffness, and reduced mobility.

Understanding the intricacies of joint replacement surgery begins with recognizing its primary goal: to alleviate pain and restore function. The decision to undergo this surgery is often made after conservative treatments, such as physical therapy, medications, and lifestyle changes, have failed to provide sufficient relief. It is a journey that requires careful consideration, as well as a deep understanding of the risks, benefits, and recovery process involved.

While the thought of surgery can be daunting, advancements in medical technology and surgical techniques have made joint replacement procedures safer and more effective than ever. Surgeons now use minimally invasive techniques, which reduce recovery time and improve outcomes. The materials used in artificial joints are also continuously evolving, with a focus on durability and biocompatibility, ensuring that these replacements can withstand the stresses of daily life for many years.

The Journey to Recovery: What to Expect

Recovery from joint replacement surgery is a journey that begins the moment you wake up from anesthesia. It's a path filled with challenges, triumphs, and learning experiences. The recovery process is multifaceted, involving not just physical healing but also mental and emotional adjustments. Knowing what to expect can help you navigate this journey with confidence and resilience.

In the immediate aftermath of surgery, the primary focus is on pain management and preventing complications such as infection or blood clots. You'll likely begin gentle movements and exercises with the guidance of a physical therapist within the first day or two after surgery. This early mobilization is crucial for promoting circulation, reducing swelling, and starting the process of regaining strength and mobility.

As you transition from the hospital to home, your recovery will shift to a more comprehensive rehabilitation phase. This period is marked by a gradual increase in physical activity and a focus on regaining independence in daily activities. You'll work closely with your healthcare team to follow a personalized rehabilitation program designed to restore strength, flexibility, and range of motion in the affected joint.

It is important to understand that recovery is not a linear process. There will be days of significant progress and others where you may feel stuck or experience setbacks. This is normal, and being prepared for these fluctuations can help you stay motivated and committed to your recovery plan. Patience and perseverance are key, as full recovery can take several months to a year, depending on the type of surgery and individual factors such as age, overall health, and the presence of any complications.

Throughout this journey, support from family, friends, and healthcare professionals is invaluable. Emotional well-being plays a crucial role in recovery, and having a strong support system can make all the difference. It's important to communicate openly with your care team about your progress, any pain or discomfort, and your emotional state. Remember, every step you take brings you closer to regaining the mobility and quality of life you seek.

By understanding what to expect after joint replacement surgery, you can prepare yourself both mentally and physically for the road ahead. With the right mindset, a commitment to rehabilitation, and a supportive network, you can navigate life post-surgery with strength and confidence, embracing the possibilities that come with a pain-free and active lifestyle.

Chapter 1:

Preparing for Surgery

Assessing the Need for Joint Replacement

Deciding to undergo joint replacement surgery is a significant step that requires careful assessment and deliberation. The first step in this process is understanding when surgery is necessary. Joint replacement is typically considered when conservative treatments—such as physical therapy, medications, injections, and lifestyle modifications—no longer provide sufficient relief from pain and limited mobility caused by conditions like osteoarthritis, rheumatoid arthritis, or significant joint trauma.

Your healthcare provider will conduct a comprehensive evaluation to determine if you're a candidate for surgery. This evaluation includes a detailed medical history, physical examination, and imaging studies such as X-rays, MRI, or CT scans. These tools help assess the extent of joint damage and determine the best course of action. A joint replacement may be recommended if the damage is severe, significantly impairs daily activities, and affects your quality of life.

Additionally, it's crucial to consider your overall health status when assessing the need for surgery. Factors such as age, weight, activity level, and the presence of other medical conditions can influence both the decision to proceed with surgery and the potential outcomes. Discussing these factors with your doctor can help you make an informed decision about whether joint replacement is the right choice for you.

Choosing the Right Surgeon and Hospital

Selecting the right surgeon and hospital is one of the most important decisions you'll make in your journey to joint replacement. Your surgeon's expertise and the quality of the hospital's facilities can significantly impact your surgery and recovery outcomes. Start by seeking a board-certified orthopedic surgeon who specializes in joint replacement. Look for a surgeon with extensive experience performing the specific type of joint replacement surgery you need, as this specialization can increase the likelihood of a successful outcome.

Research the hospital's reputation and its experience with joint replacement surgeries. Hospitals that perform a high volume of joint replacements often have better outcomes and fewer complications. Consider hospitals that are recognized as centers of excellence for orthopedic surgery, which often have dedicated teams and resources for joint replacement patients.

You can gather information about potential surgeons and hospitals through online reviews, patient testimonials, and word-of-mouth recommendations from friends, family, or your primary care physician. During your consultation with the surgeon, don't hesitate to ask questions about their experience, the surgical procedure, potential risks, and expected outcomes. Feeling comfortable and confident in your surgeon's abilities and approach is essential to your peace of mind leading up to surgery.

Pre-Surgery Physical Conditioning

Preparing your body for joint replacement surgery can positively affect your recovery and overall outcome. Physical conditioning before surgery, often referred to as "prehabilitation," aims to strengthen the muscles around the affected joint, improve cardiovascular fitness, and enhance flexibility and mobility. A well-conditioned body can better handle the physical stress of surgery and promote a smoother, faster recovery.

Your healthcare team, including a physical therapist, can design a tailored exercise program that focuses on strengthening the muscles that support your joint. For knee and hip replacements, this might include exercises that target the quadriceps, hamstrings, glutes, and core muscles. For shoulder replacements, exercises may focus on the rotator cuff and upper back muscles.

In addition to strengthening exercises, incorporating low-impact aerobic activities such as walking, swimming, or cycling can help improve your cardiovascular fitness and overall endurance. Flexibility and range-of-motion exercises are also crucial, as they can help maintain or improve the joint's movement before surgery. Remember to consult your healthcare provider before starting any new exercise program to ensure it's safe and appropriate for your condition.

Mental and Emotional Preparation

Preparing mentally and emotionally for joint replacement surgery is as important as physical preparation. Undergoing surgery can be an overwhelming experience filled with anxiety, fear, and uncertainty. Addressing these feelings before surgery can help reduce stress and promote a more positive outlook, which is beneficial for recovery.

Start by educating yourself about the surgery, recovery process, and potential challenges. Understanding what to expect can help alleviate fears and build confidence in your ability to navigate the journey ahead. Speak with your surgeon, attend pre-surgery classes, and consider joining a support group of individuals who have undergone similar procedures. Hearing about their experiences can provide valuable insights and encouragement.

It's also essential to acknowledge and address any emotional concerns you may have. Communicate openly with your family, friends, and healthcare team about your feelings and expectations. Consider relaxation techniques such as deep breathing, meditation, or mindfulness to help manage anxiety. If you're struggling with significant anxiety or depression, consulting a mental health professional can provide additional support and coping strategies.

Preparing Your Home for Post-Surgery Recovery

Creating a safe and comfortable environment at home is crucial for a smooth recovery after joint replacement surgery. Before your surgery date, take time to prepare your living space to accommodate your post-surgery needs, as this will minimize obstacles and reduce the risk of accidents during your recovery period.

Start by decluttering and rearranging furniture to create clear, wide pathways that accommodate crutches, walkers, or wheelchairs. Consider moving essential items, such as frequently used kitchenware, toiletries, and clothing, to easily accessible locations. If your bedroom is on an upper floor, you might want to set up a temporary sleeping area on the ground floor to avoid navigating stairs initially.

Installing safety aids can significantly enhance your post-surgery comfort and safety. These aids might include grab bars in the bathroom, a raised toilet seat, a shower chair, and non-slip mats. Ensure that you have a stable, comfortable chair with arms and a firm seat for sitting and getting up with ease.

Finally, consider arranging for help during the initial days or weeks after surgery. Having a family member, friend, or professional caregiver available can provide invaluable assistance with daily tasks such as meal preparation, personal hygiene, and mobility support. Being well-prepared at home can reduce stress and allow you to focus on your recovery, helping you return to your regular activities as soon as possible.

Chapter 2:

The Day of Surgery

What to Expect on the Day of Surgery

The day of your joint replacement surgery can bring a mix of emotions, from anxiety to anticipation. Knowing what to expect can help you feel more prepared and at ease. Typically, you will be asked to arrive at the hospital or surgical center a few hours before your scheduled surgery time. This allows the medical staff to complete all necessary preoperative preparations.

Upon arrival, you'll check in at the registration desk and be escorted to a preoperative area, where you'll change into a hospital gown. A nurse will take your vital signs, review your medical history, and ensure that all preoperative instructions have been followed, such as fasting or taking certain medications. You'll likely meet with your surgical team, including your surgeon, anesthesiologist, and nursing staff, who will go over the procedure again and answer any last-minute questions you may have.

You will also be asked to confirm the surgical site, and your surgeon will likely mark it with a pen to ensure accuracy. This is a routine safety measure to prevent any errors. Once all preparations are complete, you'll be given an intravenous (IV) line to administer fluids, medications, and anesthesia. At this point, you will be ready to proceed to the operating room.

Understanding Anesthesia Options

Anesthesia is a critical component of the joint replacement process, as it ensures you do not feel pain during surgery. There are several anesthesia options available, and your anesthesiologist will work with you to choose the one that best suits your needs based on your medical history, the type of joint replacement, and personal preferences.

The most common anesthesia options for joint replacement surgery include:

1. General Anesthesia: Under general anesthesia, you will be completely unconscious during the surgery. This type of anesthesia is administered through an IV or inhalation and is typically used for more extensive procedures. While it provides total pain relief and ensures you are unaware of the surgery, it may come with side effects such as grogginess, nausea, or sore throat after you wake up.

2. Regional Anesthesia: This type includes spinal or epidural anesthesia, where an anesthetic is injected near the spinal cord to numb the lower half of the body. You will remain awake during the surgery, but you will not feel any pain in the numbed area. Regional anesthesia is commonly used for hip and knee replacements and is often paired with a sedative to help you relax and potentially sleep during the procedure.

3. Local Anesthesia with Sedation: Local anesthesia involves numbing only the specific area being operated on. It's usually combined with sedatives that help you relax or fall into a light sleep. This option is less common for joint replacements but may be suitable for less invasive procedures or patients with specific medical considerations.

Your anesthesiologist will discuss the pros and cons of each option and consider any allergies, previous reactions to anesthesia, or other health conditions you may have. It's essential to communicate openly about your preferences and concerns to help the anesthesiologist tailor the anesthesia plan to your needs.

The Surgery Process: Step-by-Step

Understanding the steps involved in joint replacement surgery can help demystify the process and reduce anxiety. Here's a general outline of what happens during a typical joint replacement procedure:

1. Preparation: Once you're in the operating room, the surgical team will position you on the operating table. The anesthesiologist will administer the chosen anesthesia, and your vital signs will be continuously monitored throughout the procedure. The surgical site will be thoroughly cleaned, and sterile drapes will be placed around the area to maintain a sterile environment.

2. Incision and Exposure: The surgeon will make an incision over the affected joint. The size and location of the incision depend on the type of joint replacement and the surgical approach used. For example, a knee replacement may require a vertical incision along the front of the knee, while a hip replacement might involve an incision on the side or back of the hip. Once the incision is made, the surgeon carefully moves muscles, tendons, and other soft tissues aside to expose the joint.

3. Removal of Damaged Tissue: The surgeon will then remove the damaged bone and cartilage from the joint. This step involves precision cutting and shaping of the bone surfaces to prepare them for the new artificial joint components, or prosthesis.

4. Implantation of the Prosthesis: The artificial joint components, usually made of metal, plastic, or ceramic materials, are then fitted and secured to the prepared bone surfaces. The components are often attached using special bone cement or press-fit techniques that allow bone to grow onto the implant. The alignment and stability of the joint are carefully checked to ensure proper function and range of motion.

5. Closing the Incision: Once the prosthesis is securely in place, the surgeon will return the soft tissues to their proper positions and close the incision with sutures, staples, or surgical glue. A sterile bandage will be applied to protect the incision site.

6. Post-Surgery Protocol: After the incision is closed, you will be taken to the recovery room, where you will be monitored as you wake up from anesthesia. Pain management begins immediately, and you'll be closely observed to ensure there are no immediate complications from the surgery.

Immediate Post-Surgery Care

The first few hours after joint replacement surgery are crucial for your recovery. In the recovery room, your healthcare team will monitor your vital signs—such as heart rate, blood pressure, and oxygen levels—to ensure your body is recovering well from the anesthesia and the surgical procedure.

Pain management is a primary focus in the immediate postoperative period. You may receive pain medications through your IV line, oral medications, or a combination of both. Your pain management plan will be tailored to your needs and may include a combination of medications to control pain and reduce inflammation.

You will also be encouraged to start moving the affected joint as soon as possible, often within hours after surgery. For example, you might begin with simple ankle pumps or leg lifts in bed if you've had a knee or hip replacement. Early movement helps prevent blood clots, improves circulation, and kick-starts the rehabilitation process.

Additionally, your healthcare team will assess your ability to perform basic activities such as sitting up, transferring from the bed to a chair, and walking with the aid of crutches or a walker. Physical and occupational therapists will begin working with you to teach you how to move safely and effectively to protect your new joint and promote healing.

In the first 24 hours post-surgery, it's also crucial to monitor for any signs of complications, such as excessive bleeding, infection, or deep vein thrombosis (DVT). The healthcare team will keep a close eye on your incision site, monitor your blood pressure and heart rate, and check for any unusual symptoms.

As you stabilize and recover, you'll transition from the recovery room to a hospital room or, in some cases, to a rehabilitation facility or home. The immediate post-surgery care phase sets the foundation for a successful recovery, emphasizing the importance of pain management, mobility, and complication prevention. With the support of your healthcare team, you'll be well on your way to achieving the goals of your joint replacement surgery and regaining your quality of life.

Chapter 3:

In-Hospital Recovery

Post-Surgery Pain Management

Effective pain management is a critical aspect of your recovery process after joint replacement surgery. Properly managed pain can enhance ycur ability to participate in physical therapy, reduce the risk of complications, and promote overall healing and well-being.

Pain Medication: After surgery, your healthcare team will provide a comprehensive pain management plan tailored to your needs. This plan may include a combination of different types of medications, such as:

Opioids: Strong pain relievers that may be used for short-term pain control, especially in the first 24 to 48 hours post-surgery. Common opioids include oxycodone, hydrocodone, and morphine. While effective, opioids are typically used cautiously due to the risk of side effects, including drowsiness, constipation, and potential dependency.

Nonsteroidal Anti-Inflammatory Drugs (NSAIDs): Medications like ibuprofen or naproxen may be used to reduce inflammation and pain. These drugs are effective for managing moderate pain and can help decrease the need for opioids.

Acetaminophen: A pain reliever that can be used alone or in combination with other medications to enhance pain control without the gastrointestinal side effects associated with NSAIDs.

Nerve Blocks or Local Anesthetics: Some patients may receive a nerve block or a local anesthetic injection near the surgical site to numb the area and provide pain relief. These options can offer targeted pain control with fewer systemic side effects.

Your medical team will regularly assess your pain levels and adjust your medication regimen as needed to ensure optimal comfort. It's essential to communicate openly about your pain levels, as unmanaged pain can impede your progress and prolong your hospital stay.

Non-Medication Strategies: In addition to medications, several non-pharmacological strategies can help manage pain, such as:

Ice Therapy: Applying ice packs to the surgical site can help reduce swelling and numb the area, providing natural pain relief.

Positioning and Elevation: Proper positioning and elevation of the affected joint can minimize swelling and discomfort. Your healthcare team will guide you on how to position yourself correctly.

Relaxation Techniques: Techniques like deep breathing, meditation, or guided imagery can help reduce anxiety and improve your ability to cope with pain.

The Role of Physical Therapy

Physical therapy is a cornerstone of recovery after joint replacement surgery. It begins soon after your surgery and continues throughout your hospital stay and beyond. The primary goals of physical therapy are to restore mobility, improve strength, and promote healing.

Early Mobilization: Within hours of your surgery, a physical therapist will help you begin gentle movements and exercises. Early mobilization is critical for preventing complications like blood clots, pneumonia, and muscle stiffness. For example, after a knee or hip replacement, you might start with simple exercises such as ankle pumps, leg lifts, or bending and straightening your new joint while in bed.

Weight-Bearing and Ambulation: As you progress, you'll gradually move from sitting up in bed to standing and walking with the assistance of a walker or crutches. The therapist will teach you the proper techniques to move safely and avoid putting too much stress on your new joint. For instance, after a hip replacement, you may be instructed on how to maintain specific precautions to avoid dislocation, such as not bending the hip beyond a certain angle or twisting your leg.

Strengthening and Range of Motion Exercises: Your physical therapist will guide you through a series of exercises designed to strengthen the muscles around your new joint and improve your range of motion. These exercises are tailored to your specific surgery and recovery stage. The therapist will also provide instructions on performing these exercises at home once discharged to continue your rehabilitation.

Education and Support: Physical therapists are also educators. They will teach you how to use assistive devices, such as canes or walkers, correctly and provide tips on adapting your daily activities to protect your new joint. Additionally, they offer encouragement and motivation, helping you stay committed to your recovery goals.

Managing Potential Complications

While joint replacement surgeries are generally safe and successful, being aware of potential complications is essential to ensuring a smooth recovery. The hospital stay allows for close monitoring and prompt management of any issues that may arise.

Infection: One of the most serious complications following joint replacement surgery is infection. Signs of infection include increased redness, warmth, swelling around the incision, fever, or drainage from the surgical site. The hospital staff will take precautions to minimize the risk of infection, including using sterile techniques, administering prophylactic antibiotics, and maintaining a clean environment.

Blood Clots: Another potential complication is the formation of blood clots, or deep vein thrombosis (DVT), typically in the legs. Symptoms may include pain, swelling, or redness in the calf or thigh. To prevent blood clots, you may receive anticoagulant medications, wear compression stockings, or use a pneumatic compression device to enhance blood flow in the legs. Early mobilization and regular exercises, such as ankle pumps, also play a crucial role in preventing DVT.

Joint Stiffness or Loss of Motion: Post-surgery, some patients may experience joint stiffness or limited range of motion due to scar tissue formation or muscle weakness. Adhering to a consistent physical therapy regimen and performing prescribed exercises can help prevent these issues and promote a full recovery.

Nerve or Blood Vessel Injury: Though rare, there is a risk of nerve or blood vessel injury during surgery. This can result in numbness, weakness, or changes in sensation. The surgical team will take precautions to avoid these complications, and any symptoms should be reported immediately for evaluation and management.

Managing Other Health Conditions: If you have other chronic health conditions, such as diabetes or heart disease, these will be closely monitored during your hospital stay to prevent any adverse effects on your recovery. Maintaining stable blood sugar levels, blood pressure, and other health parameters is critical to minimizing complications.

Discharge Planning: Moving from Hospital to Home

Planning for your discharge from the hospital is a key component of your recovery process. The goal is to ensure a safe transition from hospital to home while maintaining the continuity of care and rehabilitation.

Evaluation and Assessment: Before discharge, your healthcare team will evaluate your progress and determine if you are ready to leave the hospital. They will assess your pain levels, mobility, and ability to perform basic activities such as getting in and out of bed, walking short distances, and using the bathroom. Your surgical site and overall health will also be checked to ensure no signs of complications.

Preparing for Home: Your care team will provide instructions on managing your recovery at home. This will include guidance on pain management, wound care, and recognizing signs of complications. You will receive a list of medications, including pain relievers and any other necessary prescriptions, along with detailed instructions on how and when to take them.

Physical Therapy and Follow-Up Care: Arrangements will be made for continuing physical therapy after discharge, either at home or at an outpatient facility. Your physical therapist will provide a home exercise program tailored to your needs. Regular follow-up appointments with your surgeon will also be scheduled to monitor your progress, remove sutures or staples, and address any concerns.

Home Support and Assistance: It's important to arrange for someone to help you during the initial days or weeks after returning home. This support could be a family member, friend, or professional caregiver. They can assist with daily activities such as cooking, cleaning, and personal care, allowing you to focus on your recovery.

Adapting Your Home Environment: Ensure your home is prepared for your arrival. This may include rearranging furniture to create clear pathways, installing grab bars in the bathroom, using a raised toilet seat, and setting up a sleeping area on the ground floor if needed. Having these modifications in place will help you navigate your home safely and comfortably during the recovery period.

Emotional and Psychological Support: Recovery can be challenging, and it's normal to experience a range of emotions, including frustration, anxiety, or even depression. Having a strong support network of family, friends, and healthcare professionals is crucial. Consider joining a support group or seeking counseling if needed to help you cope with the emotional aspects of recovery.

By thoroughly preparing for your discharge and adhering to your recovery plan, you can maximize your chances of a successful outcome and a return to an active, pain-free life.

Chapter 4:

The First Week Post-Surgery

Navigating the First 24 Hours

The first 24 hours after returning home from the hospital are crucial for setting the foundation for a smooth and successful recovery following joint replacement surgery. During this initial period, your primary focus should be on rest, pain management, and gradual reintroduction to mobility.

Rest and Recovery: After the stress of surgery and the journey home, it's essential to prioritize rest. Find a comfortable place to relax, ideally a designated recovery area that you prepared in advance. This space should be easy to access, with everything you need within arm's reach, including medications, water, snacks, and a phone. While rest is vital, avoid prolonged periods of immobility, which can increase the risk of complications like blood clots.

Pain Management: Managing pain effectively is crucial during the first 24 hours at home. Continue following the pain management plan provided by your healthcare team, which may include a combination of prescription medications, over-the-counter pain relievers, and non-medication strategies. Take your medications as prescribed to prevent pain from becoming severe, and monitor for any side effects such as dizziness, nausea, or constipation.

Monitoring Your Surgical Site: Keep an eye on your surgical site for any signs of infection or complications. Redness, swelling, increased warmth, drainage, or a high fever are potential signs of infection and should be reported to your healthcare provider immediately. Follow the wound care instructions provided at discharge, including keeping the incision clean and dry.

Safety Measures: Ensure that your home is set up to minimize the risk of falls or accidents. Use assistive devices such as crutches or walkers as instructed, and move slowly and carefully. Wear non-slip shoes or slippers, and avoid uneven surfaces or loose rugs that could cause you to trip.

Early Mobility: Getting Up and Moving Safely

Early mobility is a critical component of your recovery during the first week post-surgery. Moving around as soon as possible helps prevent complications such as blood clots, pneumonia, and muscle atrophy while promoting circulation and joint flexibility.

Assisted Walking: In the first week, you will likely need assistance from crutches, a walker, or a cane to help you move safely. Your physical therapist will have provided instructions on how to use these devices properly. Start by walking short distances, such as to the bathroom or kitchen, and gradually increase your activity level as you feel more comfortable and confident.

Range of Motion Exercises: Continue performing the range of motion and strengthening exercises recommended by your physical therapist. These exercises are designed to enhance flexibility, strengthen the muscles around your new joint, and promote healing. Even small movements, such as ankle pumps or gentle leg lifts, can significantly contribute to your recovery.

Adhering to Weight-Bearing Restrictions: Depending on the type of surgery and your surgeon's instructions, you may have specific weight-bearing restrictions. It is crucial to adhere to these guidelines to protect your new joint and prevent any setbacks in your recovery. Avoid putting too much weight on the affected joint until cleared by your healthcare provider.

Fall Prevention: Falls are a significant risk during the early stages of recovery. To prevent falls, use handrails when navigating stairs, avoid walking on wet or slippery surfaces, and ensure that your home is well-lit, especially at night. If you feel dizzy or unsteady, sit down and rest until you feel stable enough to continue.

Managing Pain and Swelling at Home

Effective management of pain and swelling is essential for a comfortable and successful recovery during the first week post-surgery. Swelling is a normal part of the healing process, but controlling it can help reduce pain and improve mobility.

Ice Therapy: Applying ice packs to the surgical area can help reduce swelling and numb the area, providing natural pain relief. Use ice packs for 15-20 minutes several times a day, ensuring a cloth barrier is placed between the ice pack and your skin to prevent frostbite. Ice therapy is particularly effective during the first 48 to 72 hours post-surgery when swelling is typically at its peak.

Elevation: Elevating the affected limb can help reduce swelling by promoting blood flow back toward the heart. For knee or hip replacements, try elevating the leg above heart level while lying down. Use pillows to support the leg comfortably, but avoid placing pillows directly under the knee, as this can cause stiffness and limit range of motion.

Compression: Compression garments or wraps can also help manage swelling. These garments provide gentle pressure to the area, which can reduce fluid buildup and improve circulation. Follow your healthcare provider's recommendations on the use of compression devices, such as elastic bandages or compression stockings.

Medication Adherence: Continue taking your prescribed pain medications as directed, even if you feel you can tolerate the pain. Staying ahead of the pain can make it easier to engage in physical therapy and other activities essential for recovery. If you experience any side effects or have concerns about your medication regimen, contact your healthcare provider for advice.

The Importance of Hydration and Nutrition

Proper hydration and nutrition are vital for your body's healing process after joint replacement surgery. They support tissue repair, boost your immune system, and provide the energy needed for rehabilitation.

Staying Hydrated: Drink plenty of fluids throughout the day to stay hydrated. Water is the best option, but you can also include clear broths, herbal teas, and electrolyte-replenishing drinks, especially if you are taking medications that may cause dehydration. Avoid caffeinated or sugary beverages, as they can contribute to dehydration and impede healing.

Balanced Nutrition: Eating a balanced diet rich in proteins, vitamins, and minerals is crucial for recovery. Protein helps repair tissues and build muscle, which is essential for regaining strength around the new joint. Include lean meats, poultry, fish, eggs, beans, nuts, and dairy products in your diet. Vitamins and minerals such as Vitamin C, Vitamin D, calcium, and zinc play important roles in wound healing and bone health. Incorporate a variety of fruits and vegetables, whole grains, and low-fat dairy products to ensure you receive a broad range of nutrients.

Managing Appetite Changes: It's common to experience a reduced appetite or nausea after surgery due to anesthesia, pain medications, or inactivity. To manage these changes, eat smaller, more frequent meals throughout the day. Choose easy-to-digest foods, such as soups, smoothies, and yogurt, and gradually introduce more solid foods as your appetite improves.

Preventing Constipation: Pain medications, reduced physical activity, and changes in diet can lead to constipation after surgery. To prevent this, include high-fiber foods like whole grains, fruits, and vegetables in your meals. Staying hydrated and moving regularly can also help maintain regular bowel movements. If needed, your healthcare provider may recommend a stool softener or mild laxative.

By focusing on these key areas during the first week post-surgery—navigating the first 24 hours, safely increasing mobility, managing pain and swelling, and maintaining proper hydration and nutrition—you set a strong foundation for your recovery journey. With the right strategies and support, you can maximize your healing potential and achieve a successful return to your daily activities.

Chapter 5:

Physical Therapy and Rehabilitation

Physical therapy and rehabilitation are pivotal components of recovery following knee, hip, or shoulder replacement surgery. This chapter will explore the role of physical therapy in the healing process, provide guidance on establishing an effective rehabilitation routine, offer exercises to enhance strength and flexibility, discuss tracking progress and setting goals, and cover how to adjust to using assistive devices such as crutches, walkers, and canes.

The Role of Physical Therapy in Recovery

Physical therapy (PT) is essential for a successful recovery after joint replacement surgery. The primary goals of PT are to restore function, improve strength and mobility, reduce pain, and prevent future injuries. Here's how physical therapy supports recovery:

Restoring Mobility and Function: Physical therapy helps you regain mobility in the new joint by gently encouraging range of motion and flexibility. This is particularly important for restoring normal movement patterns and enabling you to perform daily activities such as walking, climbing stairs, and dressing.

Improving Strength and Stability: Surgery can weaken the muscles surrounding the joint. PT focuses on strengthening these muscles to support the new joint, improve balance, and enhance overall stability. Stronger muscles around the joint reduce strain and decrease the risk of falls or injuries.

Reducing Pain and Inflammation: Through targeted exercises, manual therapy, and modalities such as ice, heat, or electrical stimulation, physical therapists can help manage pain and reduce swelling. This allows for more comfortable movement and promotes faster healing.

Preventing Complications: Early engagement in physical therapy helps prevent complications such as joint stiffness, muscle atrophy, blood clots, and scar tissue formation. Your physical therapist will guide you through exercises that enhance circulation and maintain muscle tone.

Personalized Recovery Plans: Each patient's recovery is unique. Physical therapists assess your specific needs, limitations, and goals to develop a personalized rehabilitation plan. This tailored approach ensures that your therapy aligns with your capabilities and recovery timeline.

Establishing a Rehabilitation Routine

Creating a consistent rehabilitation routine is crucial for optimizing your recovery. A well-structured routine should include daily exercises, rest periods, and gradual progression based on your comfort and ability. Here's how to establish an effective routine:

Consistency is Key: Aim to perform your prescribed exercises consistently, as outlined by your physical therapist. Regular exercise helps maintain progress and prevents setbacks. Establish a daily schedule that incorporates your therapy sessions and home exercises.

Start Slow and Progress Gradually: Begin with simple, low-impact exercises that promote range of motion and reduce stiffness. As you become more comfortable and your strength improves, gradually increase the intensity and duration of your exercises under the guidance of your physical therapist.

Incorporate Rest and Recovery: Balance is important in any rehabilitation routine. Allow for adequate rest between exercise sessions to prevent overexertion and fatigue. Listen to your body and avoid pushing through pain, as this can lead to injury or setbacks.

Follow Your Physical Therapist's Guidance: Your physical therapist will provide specific instructions on which exercises to perform, how often to do them, and how to progress. Follow these recommendations closely to ensure a safe and effective recovery.

Stay Motivated: Rehabilitation can be challenging, especially in the early stages. Set small, achievable goals to keep yourself motivated and focused on your progress. Celebrate milestones, such as being able to walk a certain distance or bend your knee to a specific angle.

Exercises for Strengthening and Flexibility

A key component of rehabilitation is engaging in exercises that enhance strength and flexibility around the new joint. These exercises will vary based on the type of surgery and your specific needs. Below are some common exercises for knee, hip, and shoulder replacements:

Knee Replacement Exercises:

-Quad Sets: Tighten your thigh muscles while keeping your leg straight. Hold for 5-10 seconds and release. Repeat 10-15 times. This exercise strengthens the quadriceps, which are crucial for knee stability.

-Straight Leg Raises: Lie on your back with one leg bent and the other straight. Lift the straight leg about 12 inches off the ground, hold for a few seconds, and then lower it slowly. Repeat 10-15 times for each leg.

-Heel Slides: Lie on your back and slowly slide your heel toward your buttocks while keeping your foot on the floor. Hold for a few seconds and then slide your heel back to the starting position. Repeat 10-15 times for each leg.

Hip Replacement Exercises:

-Ankle Pumps: While lying down, move your feet up and down to improve circulation and prevent blood clots. Perform this exercise for 2-3 minutes several times a day.

-Hip Abduction: While lying on your back, slowly move your leg out to the side and back to the center. Keep your leg straight and avoid rotating your hip. Repeat 10-15 times for each leg.

-Glute Squeezes: Tighten your buttocks muscles, hold for 5-10 seconds, and then release. Repeat 10-15 times. This exercise helps strengthen the gluteal muscles, which are important for hip stability.

Shoulder Replacement Exercises:

-Pendulum Exercises: Lean forward, supporting yourself with one hand on a table or chair. Let your other arm hang down and gently swing it in small circles or back and forth. Perform this exercise for 1-2 minutes several times a day.

-Shoulder Flexion: Use your unaffected arm to help lift your surgical arm forward to shoulder height. Hold for a few seconds, then slowly lower it back down. Repeat 10-15 times.

-Isometric Shoulder Exercises: While standing or sitting, press your hand against a wall or door frame without moving your arm. Hold the pressure for 5-10 seconds and then release. Repeat 10-15 times on each side.

Always perform exercises within a pain-free range and under the guidance of your physical therapist. Avoid any movements that cause discomfort or strain on the new joint.

Tracking Progress and Setting Goals

Tracking your progress and setting realistic goals are essential aspects of a successful rehabilitation journey. Regularly monitoring your achievements helps keep you motivated and allows for timely adjustments to your recovery plan.

Document Your Progress: Keep a daily log of your exercises, pain levels, and any milestones achieved. Note any changes in mobility, strength, or range of motion. This documentation helps you and your physical therapist assess your progress and make necessary adjustments to your rehabilitation plan.

Set Realistic Goals: Establish short-term and long-term goals that align with your recovery timeline. Short-term goals might include increasing your walking distance or achieving a certain range of motion. Long-term goals could involve returning to specific activities or hobbies you enjoy.

Celebrate Milestones: Acknowledge and celebrate each milestone you reach, no matter how small. Recognizing your achievements can boost your morale and reinforce your commitment to the recovery process.

Adjust Goals as Needed: Recovery from joint replacement surgery is not always linear. There may be setbacks or plateaus. Work with your physical therapist to adjust your goals and recovery plan as needed, ensuring they remain realistic and achievable.

Stay Positive and Patient: Recovery takes time, and progress may be gradual. Focus on the improvements you've made rather than comparing yourself to others or becoming discouraged by slower-than-expected progress.

Adjusting to Assistive Devices (Crutches, Walkers, Canes)

Using assistive devices like crutches, walkers, or canes is often necessary during the early stages of recovery to ensure safety and support. Learning how to use these devices correctly is essential for preventing falls and promoting optimal healing.

Selecting the Right Device: Your healthcare team will recommend the appropriate assistive device based on your specific needs, surgery type, and weight-bearing restrictions. Crutches, walkers, and canes all serve different purposes and provide varying levels of support.

-Crutches: Typically used in the early stages of recovery when non-weight-bearing or partial weight-bearing is required. Crutches provide support on both sides and help you balance while keeping weight off the surgical leg.

-Walkers: Offer more stability than crutches and are often recommended for patients who need support on both sides but can bear some weight on the surgical leg. Walkers are ideal for those recovering from hip or knee replacement surgery.

-Canes: Used when you can bear more weight on the surgical leg but still need some assistance for balance. Canes provide support on one side and are commonly used during the later stages of recovery.

Proper Use of Assistive Devices:

-Crutches: Place both crutches under your arms, gripping the handles. Move the crutches forward simultaneously, then step with your surgical leg, followed by your non-surgical leg. Keep your weight on your hands and avoid placing pressure on your armpits to prevent nerve damage.

-Walkers: Stand in the center of the walker and grip the handles firmly. Move the walker a short distance forward, then step into the walker with your surgical leg, followed by your non-surgical leg. Ensure all four walker legs are in contact with the ground before taking a step.

-Canes: Hold the cane on the side opposite your surgical leg. Move the cane and your surgical leg forward simultaneously, then step through with your non-surgical leg. The cane should move with your surgical leg to provide support and balance.

Gradual Transition: As you progress in your recovery and gain strength and stability, your physical therapist will guide you on transitioning from one assistive device to another. This may involve moving from a walker to a cane and eventually to walking independently.

Practice and Confidence: Using an assistive device may feel awkward initially, but with practice, you will gain confidence and improve your mobility. Follow your physical therapist's instructions and practice using the device in a safe environment, such as with a family member or caregiver present.

By understanding the role of physical therapy, establishing a structured rehabilitation routine, performing targeted exercises, tracking progress, setting goals, and learning to use assistive

Chapter 6:

Emotional and Mental Well-being

Recovering from joint replacement surgery involves not only physical rehabilitation but also emotional and mental healing. Adjusting to life post-surgery can be challenging, as it often comes with a range of emotions, from relief and hope to frustration and anxiety. This chapter will explore strategies for coping with post-surgery blues, maintaining a positive outlook during recovery, understanding the role of support systems, and utilizing mindfulness and stress management techniques.

Coping with Post-Surgery Blues

It is common to experience feelings of sadness, anxiety, or frustration following joint replacement surgery. These emotions, often referred to as "post-surgery blues," can be attributed to several factors, including the impact of anesthesia, pain, reduced mobility, and the stress of adjusting to a new routine. Here are some strategies to help cope with these feelings:

Acknowledge Your Emotions: Understand that it is normal to feel down or overwhelmed after surgery. Recognizing these feelings as a natural part of the recovery process can help you address them more effectively. Allow yourself to feel what you're feeling without judgment.

Communicate Your Feelings: Share your emotions with someone you trust, whether it's a family member, friend, or healthcare professional. Talking about your experiences can provide relief and help you feel less isolated. Sometimes, simply expressing your feelings out loud can lessen their intensity.

Stay Engaged with Your Recovery: Take an active role in your recovery by following your physical therapy routine and attending all follow-up appointments. Staying engaged can give you a sense of purpose and control, which can counter feelings of helplessness or despair.

Set Realistic Expectations: Recovery from joint replacement surgery is a gradual process that requires time and patience. Set small, achievable goals for yourself, and celebrate each milestone, no matter how minor it may seem. Recognizing your progress can help boost your mood and keep you motivated.

Seek Professional Help if Needed: If feelings of sadness or anxiety persist for more than a few weeks or interfere with your daily activities, consider seeking help from a mental health professional. Therapists or counselors can provide strategies to manage these emotions and offer support during this challenging time.

Staying Positive During Recovery

Maintaining a positive outlook is crucial for a successful recovery, as it can influence both your mental state and physical healing. A positive mindset can enhance your motivation, increase your resilience, and improve your overall well-being. Here are some tips for staying positive:

Focus on the Benefits of Surgery: Remind yourself why you chose to undergo joint replacement surgery in the first place. Focus on the long-term benefits, such as reduced pain, increased mobility, and improved quality of life. Visualize the activities you will be able to enjoy once you have fully recovered.

Practice Gratitude: Cultivating a sense of gratitude can shift your focus from what you have lost to what you still have. Consider keeping a gratitude journal where you write down three things you are grateful for each day. This practice can help you maintain a positive perspective and find joy in everyday moments.

Engage in Activities You Enjoy: While your mobility may be limited initially, find ways to engage in activities that bring you happiness. Whether it's reading, listening to music, watching movies, or spending time with loved ones, doing things you enjoy can lift your spirits and provide a welcome distraction from pain or discomfort.

Stay Connected with Others: Social interaction is vital for maintaining a positive outlook. Stay in touch with family and friends through phone calls, video chats, or in-person visits if possible. Sharing your recovery journey with others can provide emotional support and remind you that you are not alone.

Stay Mindful of Your Self-Talk: Pay attention to the way you talk to yourself during recovery. Replace negative self-talk with positive affirmations and constructive thoughts. Instead of thinking, "I'll never get better," try saying, "Recovery is a process, and I am making progress every day."

The Role of Support Systems (Family, Friends, Support Groups)

Having a strong support system is crucial for emotional and mental well-being during recovery. Family, friends, and support groups can provide encouragement, practical assistance, and a sense of community. Here's how to make the most of your support systems:

Lean on Family and Friends: Don't be afraid to ask for help from your loved ones. Whether it's assisting with daily tasks, providing transportation to appointments, or simply offering a listening ear, family and friends can play a significant role in your recovery. Accepting help can reduce your stress and allow you to focus on healing.

Join a Support Group: Support groups offer a platform to connect with others who are going through similar experiences. Sharing your journey with others who understand what you're going through can be incredibly validating and reassuring. Many hospitals and rehabilitation centers offer support groups for joint replacement patients, both in-person and online.

Find a Recovery Buddy: If you know someone who has undergone a similar surgery or is in the process of recovering, consider partnering up as recovery buddies. You can motivate each other, share tips and experiences, and provide mutual support during tough times.

Communicate Your Needs Clearly: Your loved ones may want to help but may not always know how. Be clear about what you need, whether it's help with physical tasks, emotional support, or just some company. Clear communication ensures that your support system can provide the most effective assistance.

Stay Open to Professional Support: In addition to personal support systems, consider seeking professional support from a counselor, therapist, or social worker. These professionals are trained to help you navigate the emotional aspects of recovery and can offer tools and strategies to cope with challenges.

Mindfulness and Stress Management Techniques

Mindfulness and stress management are essential tools for maintaining emotional balance during recovery. These techniques can help you stay grounded, reduce anxiety, and manage pain more effectively. Here are some strategies to incorporate into your daily routine:

Mindfulness Meditation: Mindfulness meditation involves focusing on the present moment without judgment. Practicing mindfulness can help you become more aware of your thoughts and emotions, allowing you to respond to them calmly rather than react impulsively. Start with just a few minutes of mindful breathing each day, gradually increasing the duration as you become more comfortable.

Deep Breathing Exercises: Deep breathing is a simple yet powerful tool for reducing stress and anxiety. Practice slow, deep breaths, inhaling through your nose, holding for a few seconds, and exhaling through your mouth. Deep breathing can calm your nervous system, reduce tension, and help you feel more centered.

Progressive Muscle Relaxation: This technique involves tensing and then relaxing different muscle groups in your body, helping to release physical tension and promote relaxation. Start from your toes and work your way up to your head, focusing on each muscle group individually. Progressive muscle relaxation can be particularly helpful for managing pain and improving sleep.

Guided Imagery: Guided imagery is a technique that involves visualizing a peaceful, calming scene or situation. This practice can help reduce stress, distract from pain, and improve mood. You can find guided imagery exercises online or create your own mental "happy place" to visit whenever you need a break from stress.

Journaling: Writing down your thoughts and feelings can be a therapeutic way to process your emotions during recovery. Journaling allows you to express yourself freely and reflect on your progress. It can also serve as a valuable tool for tracking your emotional journey and identifying patterns or triggers that may affect your mood.

Stay Physically Active Within Your Limits: Gentle physical activity, as recommended by your physical therapist, can help reduce stress, improve mood, and promote overall well-being. Even small movements, such as stretching or walking short distances, can release endorphins and boost your mood.

Practice Self-Compassion: Be kind to yourself during recovery. Understand that it's okay to have good days and bad days and that healing is a gradual process. Treat yourself with the same compassion you would offer a friend in a similar situation.

By addressing both the physical and emotional aspects of recovery, you can create a more holistic approach to healing. Coping with post-surgery blues, maintaining a positive outlook, leveraging support systems, and practicing mindfulness and stress management techniques will help you navigate the challenges of recovery with resilience and grace.

Chapter 7:

Nutrition and Healing

Nutrition plays a vital role in the recovery process after knee, hip, or shoulder replacement surgery. A balanced diet provides the body with essential nutrients that support healing, reduce inflammation, and enhance overall well-being. This chapter will discuss the importance of a balanced diet for recovery, foods that promote healing, supplements and vitamins for joint health, and the crucial role of hydration in the recovery process.

The Importance of a Balanced Diet for Recovery

A balanced diet is crucial for optimal recovery following joint replacement surgery. The body requires a variety of nutrients to repair tissues, manage inflammation, maintain muscle mass, and support overall health. Here's why a balanced diet is essential:

Supports Tissue Repair and Healing: After surgery, the body needs adequate protein, vitamins, and minerals to repair tissues, heal incisions, and rebuild muscle mass. A diet rich in lean proteins, fruits, vegetables, whole grains, and healthy fats provides these essential nutrients.

Reduces Inflammation: Some foods have anti-inflammatory properties that can help reduce swelling and pain after surgery. Incorporating these foods into your diet can enhance your recovery by minimizing discomfort and promoting healing.

Maintains Immune Function: A strong immune system is vital for preventing infections and complications post-surgery. Nutrients like vitamin C, zinc, and antioxidants support immune function and help the body ward off infections during the healing process.

Prevents Muscle Loss: Surgery and reduced mobility can lead to muscle atrophy. Consuming enough protein helps maintain muscle mass and strength, which are critical for regaining mobility and supporting the new joint.

Enhances Energy Levels: Recovery requires energy, and a balanced diet provides the necessary fuel to keep your energy levels up. Complex carbohydrates, healthy fats, and proteins are essential for sustained energy throughout the day.

Promotes Overall Well-being: Good nutrition not only supports physical recovery but also impacts mental and emotional health. Eating a variety of nutrient-dense foods can help improve mood, reduce stress, and contribute to a more positive outlook during recovery.

Foods that Promote Healing

Certain foods are particularly beneficial for promoting healing and recovery after joint replacement surgery. These foods are rich in nutrients that support tissue repair, reduce inflammation, and strengthen the immune system. Here are some of the best foods to include in your recovery diet:

1. Lean Proteins: Protein is essential for repairing tissues, maintaining muscle mass, and supporting immune function. Include sources of lean protein such as chicken, turkey, fish, eggs, tofu, beans, and low-fat dairy products. These foods provide the building blocks needed for recovery and muscle maintenance.

2. Fruits and Vegetables: Rich in vitamins, minerals, and antioxidants, fruits and vegetables play a crucial role in reducing inflammation and supporting the immune system. Focus on colorful, nutrient-dense options like berries, oranges, spinach, kale, broccoli, and bell peppers. These foods are high in vitamin C, vitamin A, and other nutrients that promote healing.

3. Whole Grains: Whole grains provide complex carbohydrates that offer sustained energy and are rich in fiber, which aids digestion. Choose whole grains like quinoa, brown rice, whole wheat bread, and oatmeal to keep your energy levels stable and support overall recovery.

4. Healthy Fats: Healthy fats are important for reducing inflammation and supporting cell health. Include sources of unsaturated fats such as avocados, nuts, seeds, olive oil, and fatty fish like salmon and mackerel, which are high in omega-3 fatty acids. Omega-3s have anti-inflammatory properties that can help reduce post-surgery swelling and pain.

5. Dairy or Fortified Alternatives: Calcium and vitamin D are crucial for bone health, especially after joint replacement surgery. Include dairy products like milk, yogurt, and cheese, or fortified plant-based alternatives like almond or soy milk. These foods provide the necessary nutrients for bone strength and healing.

6. Foods Rich in Zinc: Zinc is important for wound healing and immune function. Foods rich in zinc include lean meats, shellfish, legumes, seeds, nuts, and whole grains. Including zinc-rich foods in your diet can help speed up the healing process and reduce the risk of infection.

7. Foods High in Vitamin C: Vitamin C is essential for collagen production, which is important for wound healing and maintaining the integrity of tissues around the new joint. Citrus fruits, strawberries, bell peppers, and tomatoes are excellent sources of vitamin C.

Supplements and Vitamins for Joint Health

While a balanced diet should provide most of the nutrients needed for recovery, certain supplements and vitamins may support joint health and aid in the healing process. However, it is important to consult with your healthcare provider before starting any new supplements to ensure they are safe and appropriate for your individual needs. Here are some supplements that may benefit joint health:

1. Vitamin D: Vitamin D is crucial for calcium absorption and bone health. It also plays a role in muscle function, which is important for mobility and stability after joint replacement surgery. If you have low levels of vitamin D, a supplement may be recommended to support bone healing and overall recovery.

2. Calcium: Calcium is essential for bone health and may be particularly important if you have had hip or knee replacement surgery. A calcium supplement may be beneficial if you are not getting enough calcium from your diet, especially in the early stages of recovery when bone healing is critical.

3. Omega-3 Fatty Acids: Omega-3 supplements, such as fish oil, have anti-inflammatory properties that can help reduce joint pain and swelling. Omega-3s also support heart health, which is important for overall well-being during recovery.

4. Glucosamine and Chondroitin: These supplements are often used to support joint health and may help maintain cartilage integrity. While research on their effectiveness is mixed, some patients find them helpful for reducing joint pain and improving mobility.

5. Zinc: If you are not getting enough zinc from your diet, a supplement may support wound healing and immune function. Zinc is particularly important during the initial stages of recovery when the body is actively repairing tissues.

6. Vitamin C: A vitamin C supplement can support collagen production and tissue repair, especially if your dietary intake is insufficient. Vitamin C also has antioxidant properties that help reduce inflammation and support immune function.

Hydration and Its Role in Recovery

Hydration is a critical but often overlooked aspect of recovery after joint replacement surgery. Adequate hydration supports various bodily functions, including nutrient transport, temperature regulation, and joint lubrication. Staying well-hydrated is essential for optimal healing and overall well-being. Here's why hydration is important for recovery:

1. Aids in Nutrient Transport and Absorption: Water is necessary for transporting nutrients throughout the body and ensuring they reach the tissues that need them most. Proper hydration helps deliver essential nutrients to the surgical site, supporting tissue repair and healing.

2. Reduces the Risk of Complications: Dehydration can increase the risk of complications such as blood clots, urinary tract infections, and constipation. Staying hydrated helps maintain healthy blood flow, supports kidney function, and promotes regular bowel movements.

3. Lubricates Joints: Water plays a crucial role in maintaining joint health by keeping the synovial fluid (the lubricating fluid within the joints) at optimal levels. Proper hydration helps reduce joint stiffness and supports smooth, pain-free movement during recovery.

4. Manages Swelling and Inflammation: Hydration helps regulate body temperature and reduces inflammation by flushing out toxins and waste products from the body. Staying hydrated can help minimize post-surgery swelling and promote a more comfortable recovery.

5. Enhances Energy Levels: Dehydration can lead to fatigue, dizziness, and decreased cognitive function. Maintaining adequate hydration levels ensures that your body has the energy it needs to heal and recover efficiently.

Tips for Staying Hydrated:

-Drink Water Regularly: Aim for at least 8-10 cups (64-80 ounces) of water per day, depending on your body size, activity level, and overall health. Keep a water bottle with you throughout the day to remind you to drink regularly.

-Incorporate Hydrating Foods: Foods with high water content, such as fruits (watermelon, oranges, strawberries) and vegetables (cucumbers, lettuce, celery), can contribute to your daily hydration needs.

-Avoid Dehydrating Beverages: Limit your intake of caffeinated and alcoholic beverages, as they can have a diuretic effect and contribute to dehydration. If you consume these beverages, balance them with extra water.

-Monitor Your Hydration Status: Pay attention to signs of dehydration, such as dark urine, dry mouth, dizziness, and fatigue. Aim for light yellow urine as an indicator of adequate hydration.

By prioritizing a balanced diet, incorporating healing-promoting foods, considering appropriate supplements, and staying well-hydrated, you can support your body's recovery and enhance your overall well-being after joint replacement surgery. Proper nutrition and hydration are key components of a successful recovery, helping you return to your normal activities with strength and vitality.

Chapter 8:

Long-Term Recovery and Lifestyle Adjustments

Moving Beyond the First Few Weeks

After the initial recovery phase, which usually involves a few weeks of rest and basic rehabilitation, it's time to focus on the long-term aspects of recovery. Moving beyond the first few weeks is about gradually increasing your activity level while still protecting your body and managing any remaining pain or discomfort. It's crucial to listen to your body and avoid rushing the process. During this time, you may still experience some stiffness, swelling, or pain, but these symptoms should steadily decrease as you regain strength and mobility.

Key strategies for this phase include:

-Gradual Increase in Activity: Slowly reintroduce more activities into your daily routine. Start with light household tasks or short walks, and progressively increase the duration and intensity as you feel more comfortable.

-Continued Physical Therapy: Maintain regular physical therapy sessions, if prescribed. Your therapist will help you adapt exercises as you improve, focusing on restoring full range of motion and building strength in the muscles surrounding the joint.

-**Monitoring for Complications:** Keep an eye out for any signs of complications, such as increased swelling, redness, or severe pain, and consult your healthcare provider if you notice any of these symptoms.

Returning to Daily Activities: Tips and Techniques

Returning to daily activities is a significant milestone in your recovery journey. It requires a balance of patience and determination to ensure that you do not overexert yourself and risk setbacks.

-**Prioritize Low-Impact Activities:** Start with low-impact activities like walking, swimming, or cycling, which are easier on your joints and can help improve cardiovascular health without putting undue stress on your new joint.

-**Practice Proper Body Mechanics:** Use correct posture and body mechanics when lifting, bending, or performing any task that could strain your joint. This includes bending at the knees rather than the waist and avoiding twisting movements that can cause discomfort or damage.

-Set Realistic Goals: Break down tasks into manageable steps and set realistic goals for what you want to accomplish each week. Celebrate small victories to stay motivated.

-Use Assistive Devices if Needed: Don't hesitate to use assistive devices like canes, walkers, or grab bars if they make it easier and safer to perform daily tasks.

Understanding Long-Term Pain Management

Long-term pain management is a critical component of recovery, especially for those who continue to experience discomfort beyond the typical healing period. Pain can stem from various sources, such as inflammation, muscle weakness, or nerve sensitivity.

-Medication Management: Follow your doctor's advice regarding the use of pain medications, whether they are over-the-counter or prescribed. Be mindful of the potential for dependency or side effects, and seek alternatives when appropriate.

-Incorporate Anti-Inflammatory Diet: Continue to follow an anti-inflammatory diet rich in fruits, vegetables, whole grains, and lean proteins. Certain foods like turmeric, ginger, fatty fish, and berries can help reduce inflammation and manage pain.

-Mind-Body Techniques: Practices like mindfulness meditation, deep breathing exercises, and progressive muscle relaxation can help you manage pain by reducing stress and promoting relaxation.

-Physical Therapy and Exercise: Regular exercise can help manage pain by improving joint function and muscle strength. Work with a physical therapist to develop a safe and effective exercise plan tailored to your needs.

Adjusting to Your New Joint

Adapting to a new joint can take time, and it's normal to feel a range of emotions from excitement about improved mobility to frustration with the pace of recovery. Understanding how to adjust both physically and mentally is key to a successful long-term outcome.

-Get to Know Your New Joint: Spend time learning about your new joint and how it functions. This includes understanding any limitations and how to protect the joint during various activities.

-Embrace Lifestyle Changes: Be open to making necessary lifestyle changes to accommodate your new joint. This might include modifying your exercise routine, altering your workspace to reduce strain, or even changing how you perform daily tasks.

-Support Systems: Stay connected with your support systems, including friends, family, and healthcare professionals. Their encouragement and advice can be invaluable as you adapt to your new normal.

-Stay Positive and Patient: Remember that adjusting to a new joint is a process that takes time. Focus on the progress you've made rather than the setbacks, and be patient with yourself as you continue to heal.

Developing a Sustainable Exercise Routine

A sustainable exercise routine is crucial for maintaining joint health and overall well-being. Regular physical activity helps keep your joint flexible and strong, reduces stiffness, and improves your overall quality of life.

-Start Slow and Progress Gradually: Begin with gentle exercises, such as stretching and range-of-motion activities, and gradually increase the intensity and duration as your strength and endurance improve.

-Incorporate Strength Training: Strengthening the muscles around your joint can help stabilize and protect it. Include exercises targeting both the large muscle groups and smaller stabilizing muscles.

-Mix in Cardiovascular Activities: Low-impact cardiovascular exercises, like walking, swimming, or cycling, are great for maintaining heart health and aiding in weight management, which can reduce stress on your joints.

-Consistency is Key: Aim for a balanced routine that includes aerobic exercises, strength training, flexibility, and balance exercises. Consistency is more important than intensity; aim for at least 30 minutes of moderate activity most days of the week.

-Listen to Your Body: Pay attention to how your body responds to different exercises. If you experience pain that doesn't subside with rest or feel unusual discomfort, it's important to adjust your routine and consult with a healthcare provider if needed.

By focusing on these long-term recovery strategies and lifestyle adjustments, you can ensure a smoother transition back to daily life and maintain your joint health for years to come. Remember, recovery is a journey, and the steps you take now will lay the foundation for a healthier, more active future.

Chapter 9:

Returning to Work and Hobbies

Timing Your Return to Work

Determining the right time to return to work after a period of recovery is crucial for a smooth transition and long-term well-being. The timing will depend on various factors, including the nature of your job, the demands it places on your body, your recovery progress, and your doctor's recommendations.

-Assess Your Readiness: Before deciding to return to work, evaluate your physical and mental readiness. Consider whether you can perform your job duties comfortably and safely. If your work involves heavy lifting, prolonged standing, or repetitive motions, ensure that you have regained sufficient strength and mobility to avoid injury or setbacks.

-Consult with Your Healthcare Provider: Always seek the guidance of your healthcare provider before returning to work. They can provide a professional assessment of your recovery progress and offer recommendations on whether a full or partial return is appropriate.

-Consider a Phased Return: For many, a phased return to work can be beneficial. This might involve starting with reduced hours or lighter duties and gradually increasing your workload as your body adjusts. This approach can help prevent fatigue and reduce the risk of aggravating your condition.

-Communicate with Your Employer: Be open with your employer about your recovery status and any accommodations you might need. Many workplaces are willing to make adjustments to support employees returning from a medical leave.

Adapting Your Workspace for Comfort and safety

Creating a comfortable and safe workspace is vital for maintaining your recovery progress and preventing further injury or strain. This is particularly important if your job involves long hours of sitting, standing, or repetitive movements.

-Ergonomic Adjustments: Invest in ergonomic office equipment, such as an adjustable chair with lumbar support, a desk at the proper height, and keyboard and mouse placement that reduces strain on your wrists and shoulders. Ergonomics is key to reducing the risk of pain and injury in the workplace.

-Maintain Proper Posture: Practice good posture by keeping your back straight, shoulders relaxed, and feet flat on the floor when sitting. Avoid slouching or leaning forward, which can strain your back and neck.

-Incorporate Regular Breaks and Movement: Taking regular breaks to stand up, stretch, and move around can help prevent stiffness and reduce the risk of developing pain. Consider using a timer to remind yourself to take short breaks throughout the day.

-Consider Assistive Devices: Depending on your needs, using assistive devices like a standing desk, footrest, or wrist supports can enhance comfort and reduce strain. Speak with an occupational therapist for personalized recommendations.

Resuming Hobbies and Activities

Returning to your hobbies and favorite activities is an essential part of feeling like yourself again and maintaining a balanced, fulfilling life. However, it's important to approach this process with caution and gradual reintroduction to avoid overexertion.

-Start with Low-Impact Activities: Begin with low-impact hobbies that don't place excessive stress on your body. For example, instead of running, you might start with walking or swimming, which are gentler on the joints.

-Listen to Your Body: Pay attention to any pain or discomfort that arises when resuming an activity. If you feel pain beyond mild discomfort, it's a sign to slow down or take a break.

-Modify Activities as Needed: Adapt your hobbies to accommodate any physical limitations or discomfort. For instance, if gardening, consider using raised beds or gardening stools to reduce the need for bending and kneeling.

-Gradual Progression: Just as with returning to work, reintroduce hobbies gradually. Increase the duration and intensity slowly over time to allow your body to adapt without causing injury.

The Importance of Gradual Reintegration

Gradual reintegration into work and hobbies is key to a successful recovery. Pushing yourself too hard, too soon can lead to setbacks, increased pain, or injury, which can prolong your recovery.

-Set Realistic Expectations: Understand that returning to your previous level of activity may take time. Set achievable goals and celebrate small milestones to maintain motivation and avoid frustration.

-Monitor Your Recovery: Keep track of your recovery progress by noting any changes in pain, mobility, or strength. Use this information to adjust your activities as needed and share updates with your healthcare provider.

-Stay Flexible and Patient: Be prepared to adjust your plans based on how you feel. Recovery is not always a linear process, and there may be days when you need to rest more or reduce your activity level.

-Maintain a Balanced Routine: Ensure your routine includes time for work, hobbies, rest, and self-care. A balanced approach will help you avoid burnout and support a sustainable recovery.

By carefully planning your return to work and hobbies, and making necessary adjustments to your environment and activities, you can ensure a smoother transition and continued progress in your recovery journey. Remember that patience and flexibility are essential components of long-term success.

Chapter 10:

Preventing Future Joint Problems

Understanding the Lifespan of Your New Joint

Your new joint, whether from surgery or other forms of joint treatment, has a lifespan that can vary depending on several factors, including the type of joint replacement, your age, activity level, and overall health. On average, most joint replacements, such as hip and knee replacements, can last 15 to 20 years or more with proper care.

-Material and Type of Joint Replacement: Modern joint replacements are made from durable materials such as metal, plastic, and ceramic. The type of material used can affect the joint's longevity. For example, ceramic joints tend to wear down less quickly than metal or plastic joints.

-Your Age and Activity Level: Younger, more active individuals may experience more wear and tear on their new joints, potentially shortening their lifespan. Conversely, older individuals or those with lower activity levels may find their joint replacements last longer.

-Adherence to Recovery and Maintenance Protocols: Following your healthcare provider's recommendations for rehabilitation, avoiding high-impact activities, and maintaining a healthy lifestyle can all contribute to maximizing the lifespan of your new joint.

Avoiding High-Impact Activities

High-impact activities can place undue stress on your new joint, potentially accelerating wear and tear and increasing the risk of injury or complications. Understanding which activities to avoid and how to modify your exercise routine is crucial for protecting your joint.

-**What to Avoid:** High-impact activities such as running, jumping, heavy lifting, and high-intensity sports like basketball or tennis should be avoided unless specifically cleared by your healthcare provider. These activities can cause excessive pressure and shock to the joint, leading to faster wear or damage.

-**Low-Impact Alternatives:** Focus on low-impact exercises that provide cardiovascular benefits without putting stress on your joints. Walking, swimming, cycling, and yoga are excellent alternatives that can help maintain fitness and joint mobility while minimizing risk.

-Modifying Existing Activities: If you have a favorite high-impact activity, consult with a physical therapist to explore ways to modify the exercise to make it safer for your new joint. For example, switching from running to using an elliptical machine can provide a similar workout with less impact.

Maintaining Joint Health Through Diet and Exercise

A healthy diet and regular exercise are essential components of joint health, helping to maintain a healthy weight, reduce inflammation, and strengthen the muscles around your joints.

-Anti-Inflammatory Diet: Continue to follow an anti-inflammatory diet rich in fruits, vegetables, whole grains, lean proteins, and healthy fats. Foods such as leafy greens, berries, fatty fish, nuts, and seeds are particularly beneficial for reducing inflammation and supporting joint health.

-Hydration: Staying well-hydrated helps maintain the lubrication of your joints, which is vital for smooth movement and reducing wear and tear.

-Regular Targeted Exercise: Incorporate exercises that focus on flexibility, strength, and endurance. Strengthening the muscles around your joint provides better support and stability, which can reduce strain on the joint itself. Flexibility exercises like stretching or yoga can help maintain a good range of motion.

-Weight Management: Maintaining a healthy weight is crucial for joint health. Excess weight places additional stress on your joints, particularly weight-bearing joints like the hips and knees, increasing the risk of wear and tear and joint problems.

Regular Check-Ups and Monitoring

Regular check-ups with your healthcare provider are vital for ensuring the ongoing health of your new joint and preventing future problems. These appointments allow your doctor to monitor the condition of the joint, assess your overall recovery progress, and make any necessary adjustments to your care plan.

-Routine Follow-Up Appointments: Attend all scheduled follow-up appointments with your orthopedic surgeon or healthcare provider. These visits are important for checking the joint's alignment, function, and overall condition, and for discussing any concerns you may have.

-Imaging Tests: Periodic imaging tests, such as X-rays or MRIs, may be recommended to assess the condition of your joint replacement and detect any signs of wear, loosening, or other issues that may need attention.

-Early Detection of Problems: Regular monitoring helps in the early detection of any problems, such as joint loosening or infection, which can often be managed more effectively when caught early.

-Open Communication: Keep an open line of communication with your healthcare provider. If you experience new or worsening pain, swelling, or other symptoms, don't wait until your next appointment—contact your doctor promptly.

By understanding the lifespan of your new joint, avoiding high-impact activities, maintaining joint health through diet and exercise, and adhering to regular check-ups and monitoring, you can help prevent future joint problems and ensure the long-term success of your joint replacement or treatment. Taking these proactive steps will allow you to enjoy a more active and pain-free life, supporting overall well-being and mobility.

Chapter 11:

Dealing with Setbacks

Identifying and Managing Complications

While most recoveries proceed smoothly, setbacks and complications can sometimes occur, delaying progress or causing new challenges. Identifying and managing these complications early can prevent more serious issues and ensure a quicker return to recovery.

-Common Complications: Potential complications after joint surgery or treatment can include infections, blood clots, joint stiffness, swelling, and pain. Other issues may involve the loosening or dislocation of the joint replacement, especially if the joint is overused or improperly cared for.

-Recognizing Symptoms: It is crucial to be aware of the signs and symptoms of complications. Redness, increased swelling, warmth around the joint, fever, or unusual pain could indicate an infection. Persistent pain, a clicking sensation, or a feeling that the joint is "giving way" might suggest a problem with the joint itself.

-Immediate Steps: If you suspect a complication, it's important to take immediate steps. Rest the affected joint, apply ice to reduce swelling, and elevate it if possible. Avoid any activities that might exacerbate the issue until you can consult with a healthcare professional.

When to Seek Medical Advice

Knowing when to seek medical advice is vital for managing setbacks effectively. Prompt consultation with a healthcare provider can make a significant difference in addressing complications early and avoiding more severe problems.

-Signs to Watch For: Seek medical advice if you experience persistent pain, swelling, or redness that doesn't improve with home care, fever or chills, increased drainage or foul-smelling discharge from a surgical site, or a sudden loss of function or stability in the joint.

-Understanding Your Threshold: Everyone's recovery journey is unique, and what may be a minor setback for one person could be a significant issue for another. Trust your instincts and reach out to your healthcare provider if you feel something isn't right, even if it seems minor.

-Scheduled Follow-Ups: Even outside of emergencies, maintain regular communication with your healthcare provider through scheduled follow-up appointments. These check-ins are crucial for monitoring recovery and making necessary adjustments to your care plan.

Coping with Slow Progress or Regression

Recovery is not always a linear process, and it's common to experience periods of slow progress or even regression. These moments can be frustrating and disheartening, but there are strategies to help you cope and stay motivated.

-Set Realistic Expectations: Understand that recovery timelines can vary widely.

While some people may recover quickly, others may need more time, especially if there are complications or other health conditions involved. Setting realistic expectations can help manage frustration.

-Celebrate Small Wins: Focus on small improvements rather than the overall timeline. Whether it's a slight increase in range of motion or a reduction in pain, celebrating these milestones can help maintain a positive outlook.

-Adjust Your Plan: Work with your healthcare provider to adjust your recovery plan as needed. This might involve altering your exercise routine, changing medications, or adding new therapies to address specific challenges.

-Mental and Emotional Support: Dealing with slow progress or setbacks can be mentally and emotionally taxing. Consider seeking support from friends, family, or a professional counselor to help you navigate these feelings. Joining a support group of others who are going through similar experiences can also provide comfort and motivation.

The Role of Second Surgeries or Revisions

In some cases, a second surgery or revision might be necessary to address complications or improve joint function. While this can feel like a setback, revisions can also offer a path forward to better health and mobility.

-Understanding Revisions: Revision surgery is performed to replace or repair a joint replacement that has failed, become loose, or caused ongoing pain or dysfunction. This procedure can be more complex than the initial surgery and requires a skilled orthopedic surgeon with experience in revisions.

-When Revisions Are Needed: Not all setbacks require surgery, but if conservative treatments fail to resolve issues like persistent pain, instability, or infection, a revision may be recommended. Your surgeon will perform a thorough evaluation, including imaging tests and possibly blood work, to determine the best course of action.

-Preparing for Revision Surgery: Preparing for a revision surgery involves similar steps to the initial surgery, including preoperative testing, optimizing your health, and discussing any concerns or questions with your surgeon. It's essential to have realistic expectations about recovery, which might take longer than the initial surgery.

-Recovery After Revision: Recovery from a revision surgery can be more challenging due to increased surgical complexity and the condition of the joint and surrounding tissues. Adherence to rehabilitation protocols, maintaining a healthy lifestyle, and being proactive about any signs of complications are crucial for a successful recovery.

By understanding potential setbacks, knowing when to seek help, coping with slow progress, and being open to the possibility of further surgery, you can navigate the complexities of recovery more effectively. Each setback is an opportunity to reassess, adapt, and continue on the path toward improved health and mobility.

Chapter 12:

Success Stories and Testimonial

Real-Life Experiences of Joint Replacement Patients

earing about the experiences of others who have undergone joint replacement surgery can provide invaluable insight and encouragement for new patients. The journey through surgery and recovery is unique to each individual, but the common thread of perseverance, adaptation, and eventual triumph offers inspiration to all.

-Patient A: Overcoming the Fear of Surgery: Sarah, a 58-year-old avid gardener, faced knee replacement surgery after years of debilitating arthritis. Initially, she was fearful of the surgery and the potential for complications. However, her determination to return to her beloved garden motivated her to follow her surgeon's advice carefully. Post-surgery, Sarah adhered strictly to her physical therapy regimen, and within six months, she was back to tending her garden with minimal discomfort. Her experience taught her the importance of trusting her medical team and staying positive throughout the recovery process.

-Patient B: A Journey Back to Sports: Tom, a 45-year-old former high school athlete, underwent a hip replacement after an old sports injury deteriorated over time. His goal was to return to playing tennis, which he loved. Through a combination of personalized rehabilitation exercises and consistent support from his physical therapist, Tom gradually regained his strength and agility. A year after surgery, he was back on the tennis court, playing at a level he hadn't thought possible. Tom's story emphasizes the value of setting specific recovery goals and being patient with the healing process.

-Patient C: Finding New Joy in Movement: Maria, 72, underwent shoulder replacement surgery after years of chronic pain that limited her ability to perform daily tasks. Post-surgery, she focused on regaining her independence. She followed a tailored physical therapy program, gradually building strength and range of motion. Six months later, Maria discovered a newfound love for water aerobics, a low-impact exercise that kept her active without stressing her new joint. Her story highlights the importance of exploring new activities and hobbies post-recovery.

Lessons Learned and Advice for New Patients

The lessons learned from these real-life experiences provide practical advice for new patients facing joint replacement surgery.

-Follow Your Rehabilitation Plan: Consistent adherence to a rehabilitation plan is crucial for a successful recovery. Many patients found that sticking to their prescribed physical therapy regimen, even when it was challenging, made a significant difference in their outcomes.

-Stay Patient and Positive: Recovery can be a long and sometimes frustrating process. Patients frequently mentioned the importance of maintaining a positive mindset and being patient with their bodies as they heal. Recovery doesn't happen overnight, and setbacks are normal, but a positive attitude can make the journey smoother.

-Communicate with Your Healthcare Team: Open communication with your healthcare providers is essential. Don't hesitate to ask questions or express concerns, whether it's about pain management, exercise, or any other aspect of your recovery. Your medical team is there to support you and ensure you have the best outcome possible.

-Build a Support Network: Having a strong support network of family, friends, or a support group of other joint replacement patients can provide emotional support and practical assistance. Sharing experiences with others who understand what you're going through can be incredibly comforting.

Inspiring Stories of Recovery and Triumph

Beyond the physical recovery, many patients experience profound emotional and psychological benefits from their joint replacement surgery. These inspiring stories of recovery and triumph show the transformative power of this journey.

-Patient D: From Pain to Passion: James, a 65-year-old retired teacher, had always dreamed of traveling after retirement, but his severe hip pain made it difficult to walk even short distances. After his hip replacement, James not only regained mobility but also discovered a passion for hiking. He has since traveled to several national parks, tackling trails he once thought impossible. His story is a testament to the idea that life after surgery can be filled with new adventures and passions.

-Patient E: Redefining Possibilities: Carol, a 50-year-old office worker, faced a double knee replacement. Before her surgery, she worried she might never be able to return to her active lifestyle. However, with a focus on recovery and support from her family, Carol not only returned to her normal activities but also took up cycling. She now participates in charity bike rides and has become a mentor for others considering joint replacement. Carol's journey shows that joint replacement can open doors to new possibilities and community engagement.

-Patient F: A New Lease on Life: Richard, a 70-year-old grandfather, underwent shoulder replacement surgery after decades of pain from an old injury. Post-surgery, he was able to play catch with his grandchildren for the first time. His renewed ability to participate in family activities brought immense joy to his life, proving that joint replacement can significantly enhance one's quality of life and strengthen family bonds.

These stories remind us that while joint replacement surgery is a significant undertaking, it also offers a pathway to renewed vitality, activity, and joy. Every patient's journey is different, but the shared experiences of overcoming fear, setting new goals, and finding joy in movement can provide hope and motivation for those facing their own recovery journey.

Chapter 13:

Frequently Asked Questions

Common Concerns Before and After Surgery

Undergoing joint replacement surgery is a significant decision, and it's natural to have many questions and concerns both before and after the procedure.

Here are some of the most common concerns raised by patients:

Pre-Surgery Concerns:

-What are the risks of surgery? Patients often worry about the risks associated with joint replacement surgery, including infection, blood clots, and anesthesia complications. Understanding these risks and discussing them with your surgeon can help you make an informed decision.

-How long will recovery take? Recovery time can vary depending on the type of surgery, the patient's overall health, and adherence to the rehabilitation plan. Most patients start to see significant improvements within 6 to 12 weeks, but complete recovery can take several months to a year.

-Will I experience a lot of pain after surgery? Post-operative pain is a common concern. Pain management is an important part of recovery, and your healthcare team will provide medications and other strategies to help control pain.

Post-Surgery Concerns:

-How do I know if my recovery is on track? It's common to worry about the progress of your recovery. Regular follow-up appointments with your surgeon or physical therapist will help monitor your progress and address any concerns.

-What activities will I be able to do? Many patients wonder about their activity levels post-surgery. Generally, low-impact activities such as walking, swimming, and cycling are encouraged. High-impact activities should be discussed with your healthcare provider.

-What if I experience a setback? Setbacks can happen, but they don't mean failure. If you experience increased pain, swelling, or other symptoms, contact your healthcare provider promptly for advice.

Answers from Medical Experts

To provide clarity and reassurance, here are answers from medical experts to some of the most frequently asked questions:

-What should I do to prepare for surgery?

Preparation involves several steps, including pre-operative testing, meeting with your surgical team, and preparing your home for post-surgery recovery. It's important to stay as active as possible before surgery to maintain muscle strength and flexibility, which can aid in recovery.

-How long will I stay in the hospital after surgery?

The hospital stay usually ranges from 1 to 3 days, depending on the type of surgery and the patient's overall health. Some patients may be discharged the same day, especially with advancements in surgical techniques and post-operative care.

-What are the signs of complications I should watch for?

Signs of complications include excessive swelling, increased pain, redness, warmth around the surgical site, fever, or any unusual symptoms. If you notice any of these signs, it's important to contact your healthcare provider immediately.

-How soon can I drive after surgery?

Driving is typically not recommended until you are off pain medications and can safely operate a vehicle without restriction. This can take several weeks, depending on the type of surgery and your recovery progress. Your surgeon will provide specific guidance based on your situation.

-Will I need assistance at home after surgery?

Yes, you will likely need some assistance with daily activities such as bathing, dressing, and meal preparation during the first few weeks post-surgery. Arranging for help from family, friends, or a professional caregiver is advisable.

Tips for a Smooth Recovery

A successful recovery from joint replacement surgery depends on several factors, including adherence to your rehabilitation plan and making necessary lifestyle adjustments. Here are some expert tips to help ensure a smooth recovery:

-Follow Your Rehabilitation Plan: Attend all scheduled physical therapy sessions and follow the exercise plan provided by your therapist. Rehabilitation is crucial for regaining strength, flexibility, and function in your new joint.

-Manage Pain Effectively: Use pain medications as prescribed and communicate with your healthcare provider if your pain is not well-controlled. Effective pain management is key to maintaining mobility and participating in rehabilitation.

-Maintain a Healthy Diet: Eating a balanced diet rich in protein, vitamins, and minerals supports healing and recovery. Staying hydrated is also important for overall health and joint function.

-Avoid High-Impact Activities: Protect your new joint by avoiding high-impact activities such as running, jumping, and heavy lifting. Focus on low-impact exercises that promote joint health and mobility.

-Keep Your Follow-Up Appointments: Regular follow-up appointments allow your healthcare provider to monitor your recovery progress and address any issues early. These check-ins are vital for long-term success.

-Listen to Your Body: Pay attention to how your body feels during recovery. If you experience increased pain, swelling, or discomfort, take a break and consult your healthcare provider if needed.

-Stay Positive and Patient: Recovery can be a slow process, and setbacks are normal.

Staying positive, setting realistic goals, and celebrating small milestones can help keep you motivated.

By addressing common concerns, providing expert answers, and offering practical tips, this chapter aims to empower you with the knowledge and confidence needed for a successful recovery journey. Remember, every recovery is unique, and staying informed and proactive can make all the difference in achieving the best possible outcome.

Recommended Products for Recovery

Using the right products can make the recovery process smoother and more comfortable. Here are some recommended products that can assist in your recovery:
-Ice Packs and Cold Therapy Systems: These are essential for reducing swelling and

managing pain post-surgery. Reusable ice packs or cold therapy machines that provide continuous cold therapy can be particularly helpful.

-Joint Support Pillows: Specially designed pillows for knee or hip support can provide comfort while sleeping and reduce strain on the new joint.

-Mobility Aids: Items such as walkers, crutches, and canes can help you move safely during the initial stages of recovery. Make sure to choose a mobility aid that fits your specific needs and consult with your physical therapist for recommendations.

-Compression Stockings: These are often recommended to reduce swelling and prevent blood clots after surgery. Be sure to follow your surgeon's instructions on how long to wear them.

-Rehabilitation Tools: Resistance bands, balance boards, and pedal exercisers can help strengthen muscles around the joint and improve range of motion as you progress in your rehabilitation.

Contact Information for National Organizations and Support Services

Several national organizations provide resources, support, and education to individuals undergoing joint replacement surgery. Here is a list of some key organizations:

-The American Academy of Orthopaedic Surgeons (AAOS): Offers extensive resources on joint replacement surgery, including patient education materials, videos, and links to finding an orthopedic surgeon.

- Website: www.aaos.org

-The Arthritis Foundation: Provides information on arthritis treatment, including joint replacement, and offers support through various programs and events.

- Website: www.arthritis.org

- Helpline: 1-800-283-7800

-The National Institute of Arthritis and Musculoskeletal and Skin Diseases (NIAMS): Part of the National Institutes of Health, NIAMS offers comprehensive information on joint replacement surgery and arthritis-related conditions.
  - Website: www.niams.nih.gov

-The Joint Replacement Network (JRN): A network offering resources, support, and connections to professionals specializing in joint replacement.
  - Website: www.jointreplacement.org

-Local and Regional Support Services: Many hospitals and clinics offer local support groups or educational seminars for joint replacement patients. Check with your healthcare provider or local community center for resources available in your area.

By leveraging these resources, you can gain a deeper understanding of joint replacement surgery, connect with a supportive community, and access tools that will aid in your recovery. Remember, education and support are key components of a successful recovery journey, so don't hesitate to reach out and take advantage of the resources available to you.

Conclusion

Reflecting on the Journey

Embarking on the journey of joint replacement surgery is no small feat. It involves facing fears, making difficult decisions, and committing to a path of healing that requires both physical and emotional strength. For many, the road to recovery is filled with both challenges and triumphs. Reflecting on this journey, it's essential to acknowledge the courage it takes to confront chronic pain and the perseverance required to regain mobility and improve quality of life. Whether you are at the beginning of your journey or well into your recovery, remember that every step forward is a testament to your resilience and determination.

Throughout this book, we've explored various aspects of the joint replacement experience, from preparing for surgery and managing pain to embracing a new lifestyle and preventing future joint issues. Each chapter has aimed to provide you with the knowledge, tools, and encouragement needed to navigate this process confidently. Your journey is unique, but you are not alone—many have walked this path before you, and countless resources are available to support you every step of the way.

Looking Forward to a Pain-Free Future

As you move forward, envision the pain-free future that motivated your decision to undergo joint replacement surgery. A future where you can engage in activities you love, spend quality time with loved ones, and pursue hobbies without the constant shadow of pain. For many, joint replacement is a transformative experience that opens up new possibilities, restores independence, and improves overall well-being.

It's important to set realistic expectations for your recovery while maintaining hope for what's possible. Many patients find that with time and commitment, they can return to or even surpass their pre-surgery levels of activity. Celebrate each milestone, no matter how small, and keep your eyes on the long-term benefits that joint replacement can bring. Whether it's playing with grandchildren, walking in the park, or simply performing daily tasks with ease, a pain-free future is within reach.

Final Tips for a Successful Recovery

As you conclude this chapter in your recovery journey, here are some final tips to help ensure your continued success:

1.**Stay Active Within Limits:** Engaging in regular, low-impact exercise is crucial for maintaining joint health and overall fitness. Activities like walking, swimming, and cycling can strengthen muscles and improve joint flexibility without placing undue stress on your new joint.

2.**Listen to Your Body:** Pay close attention to how your body feels during and after activities. Pain, swelling, or discomfort can indicate that you are overdoing it. Rest when needed and gradually increase your activity level as recommended by your healthcare provider.

3.Maintain a Healthy Diet: A balanced diet rich in anti-inflammatory foods can support joint health and overall recovery. Staying hydrated and consuming a variety of nutrients will help you heal faster and maintain energy levels.

4.Stay Engaged with Your Healthcare Team: Regular follow-ups with your surgeon, primary care physician, and physical therapist are vital for monitoring your progress and addressing any concerns. Don't hesitate to reach out to your medical team with questions or for advice on managing your recovery.

5.Embrace a Positive Mindset: Recovery is as much a mental journey as it is a physical one. Maintaining a positive outlook and staying motivated can greatly influence your recovery. Remember that setbacks are normal and can be overcome with patience and persistence.

6.Build a Support Network: Whether through family, friends, support groups, or online communities, having a network of people who understand your experience can provide emotional support, practical advice, and encouragement.

7.Educate Yourself Continuously: Keep learning about your condition, recovery techniques, and lifestyle adjustments that can enhance your quality of life. Staying informed empowers you to make the best decisions for your health.

Your journey to recovery is a personal one, marked by both challenges and triumphs. By staying proactive, informed, and supported, you can look forward to a future filled with greater mobility, less pain, and renewed opportunities to enjoy life to the fullest. Remember, you have the strength to overcome obstacles and the resources to guide you through each phase of your recovery. Here's to your continued health and a pain-free future!

Appendices

The appendices provide additional tools and information to support your journey through joint replacement surgery and recovery. These resources are designed to be practical and user-friendly, helping you better understand medical terminology, stay organized, and manage your recovery more effectively.

Glossary of Medical Terms

Understanding the medical terminology associated with joint replacement surgery can be overwhelming. This glossary aims to clarify some of the common terms you may encounter:

-Arthroplasty: Surgical repair or replacement of a joint.

-Cartilage: A flexible, rubbery tissue that covers the ends of bones in joints, providing cushioning and reducing friction.

-Cemented Prosthesis: A type of joint implant that is secured in place with surgical cement.

-Debridement: The surgical removal of damaged tissue or foreign objects from a wound.

-DVT (Deep Vein Thrombosis): A condition where blood clots form in deep veins, often in the legs, which can be a risk after surgery.

-Osteoarthritis: A degenerative joint disease characterized by the breakdown of cartilage, leading to pain and stiffness.

-Partial Knee Replacement: A surgical procedure where only a portion of the knee joint is replaced.

-Physical Therapy: A treatment method focused on improving movement, strength, and function through exercises and manual therapy.

-Prosthesis: An artificial device used to replace a missing body part, such as a joint.

-Revision Surgery: A procedure performed to replace or repair a joint implant that has failed or worn out.

-Synovial Fluid: A thick fluid found in joint cavities that reduces friction between the articular cartilage of synovial joints during movement.

-Total Hip Replacement: A surgical procedure where the entire hip joint is replaced with an artificial implant.

-Uncemented Prosthesis: A type of joint implant that allows natural bone growth to secure the implant in place without the use of cement.

Sample Exercise Routines

Physical therapy and exercise are critical components of recovery after joint replacement surgery. Here are some sample exercise routines that may be recommended by your physical therapist:

Early Post-Operative Exercises:

-**Ankle Pumps:** Lie on your back and move your ankles up and down to improve circulation and prevent blood clots.

-**Quad Sets:** Tighten the muscles on the top of your thigh, hold for 5 seconds, and then relax. This helps strengthen the quadriceps muscles.

-**Heel Slides:** Lie on your back and slowly slide your heel towards your buttocks, then back to the starting position. This helps improve knee flexibility.

Mid-Stage Recovery Exercises:

-**Straight Leg Raises:** Lie on your back with one knee bent and the other leg straight. Lift the straight leg to the height of the bent knee, hold for a few seconds, and then lower it back down.

-**Seated Knee Flexion:** Sit in a chair and gently bend your knee as far as you can, hold for a few seconds, then return to the starting position. This exercise helps improve knee range of motion.

 -**Stationary Bicycling:** Use a stationary bike with low resistance to improve joint flexibility and cardiovascular endurance.

Advanced Recovery Exercises:

 -**Mini Squats:** Stand with your feet shoulder-width apart and slowly lower your body into a squat position, keeping your knees behind your toes. Return to the starting position and repeat.

 -**Step-Ups:** Use a step or a sturdy platform to step up and down, alternating legs. This exercise helps strengthen the muscles around the hip and knee joints.

 -**Balance Exercises:** Stand on one leg while holding onto a chair or countertop for support. This helps improve balance and stability.

Pain Management Tracker

Tracking your pain levels and the effectiveness of pain management strategies can help you and your healthcare team make informed decisions about your care. Use this pain management tracker to record your pain levels, medication use, and other interventions:

Date	Time	Pain Level (0-10)	Medications Taken	Non-Medication Interventions	Notes (Activities, Triggers)
01/01/2024	8:00 AM	4	Acetaminophen 500 mg	Ice pack, Rest	Pain after morning walk
01/01	12:00	6	Ibupr	Eleva	Pain

/2024	PM		ofen 200 mg	tion, Heat Ther apy	incre ased after lunch

Meal Planning for Recovery

Proper nutrition is vital for healing and recovery after surgery. A well-balanced diet rich in anti-inflammatory foods can promote joint health and overall recovery. Here is a sample meal plan for a week to support recovery:

Breakfast:
 -Day 1: Oatmeal with berries, walnuts, and a drizzle of honey
 -Day 2: Scrambled eggs with spinach, tomatoes, and whole-grain toast
 -Day 3: Greek yogurt with honey, chia seeds, and sliced almonds

Lunch:

-**Day 1:** Quinoa salad with chickpeas, cucumber, cherry tomatoes, and a lemon-tahini dressing

-**Day 2:** Grilled chicken breast with steamed broccoli and brown rice

-**Day 3:** Lentil soup with a side of mixed greens salad

Dinner:

-**Day 1:** Baked salmon with roasted sweet potatoes and asparagus

-**Day 2:** Turkey stir-fry with bell peppers, snap peas, and a ginger-garlic sauce

-**Day 3:** Vegetable lasagna with a side of garlic bread

Snacks:

-**Day 1:** Apple slices with almond butter

-**Day 2:** Hummus with carrot and cucumber sticks

-**Day 3:** Cottage cheese with pineapple chunks

Surgery and Recovery Checklist

A checklist can help ensure that you are prepared for surgery and equipped for a smooth recovery. Here is a comprehensive surgery and recovery checklist:

Pre-Surgery Preparation:
 -Complete all pre-operative testing (blood tests, EKG, etc.)
 -Meet with your surgeon to discuss the procedure and recovery expectations
 -Arrange for transportation to and from the hospital
 -Prepare your home for recovery (remove tripping hazards, set up a recovery area)
 -Gather necessary supplies (medications, mobility aids, ice packs)

Post-Surgery Essentials:
-Follow all post-operative care instructions provided by your surgeon
-Take prescribed medications as directed
-Attend all scheduled follow-up appointments and physical therapy sessions

-Monitor for signs of complications (increased pain, swelling, fever) and contact your healthcare provider if necessary
-Use mobility aids as needed to prevent falls and promote safe movement
-Maintain a healthy diet and stay hydrated to support healing

By utilizing these appendices, you can enhance your understanding of the medical process, stay organized during recovery, and make informed decisions that contribute to a successful outcome. Remember, preparation and proactive management are key to navigating your joint replacement journey with confidence.

Made in the USA
Middletown, DE
19 September 2024